# CANCER PREVENTION AND RISK FACTORS

## Understanding the Causes of Cancer and How to Lower Your Risk

Watson L. Felix

ISBN: 9798850376840

**DEDICATION**

This book is dedicated to God, my beloved family, whose unconditional love and support have been a source of infinite inspiration and strength. To my parents, my siblings, my husband, and my children—you are the reason for this book. Thank you for everything.

# TABLE OF CONTENTS

**INTRODUCTION**

This book aims to help readers develop an understanding of the risk factors associated with cancer, and the steps to take to reduce the risk of developing cancer. It provides readers with an up-to-date overview of cancer prevention, screening strategies, diagnosis, and treatment. It explains the various causes of cancer, how to detect it early, and how to treat and manage it. Through its comprehensive discussion of the many factors contributing to the risk of developing cancer, this book provides invaluable insight into identifying and managing preventive measures, both individually and at the community and population levels.

The book begins by addressing the history and epidemiology of different types of cancer. It addresses the economic burden associated with the treatment of cancer, as well as discusses advances in current and upcoming treatments. It also explores the most effective preventive strategies for all major types of cancer. This section explores lifestyle and environmental factors as well as dietary and nutritional strategies, along with citations from leading medical and scientific research.

The remaining sections delve further into many of the controversies surrounding current cancer screening practices, genetic susceptibility, targeted cancer preventive approaches, early detection, and effective treatments. It also discusses important implications of current legislation, clinical guidelines, and media coverage. Crucially, this book keeps its finger firmly on the pulse of current cancer research and thinking.

Throughout this book, the authors provide even-handed yet incisive critiques of ongoing debates between researchers and medical practitioners, allowing readers to develop their own, informed opinions on the matter. Summaries of salient points in each chapter are provided for easy reference. This book serves as an invaluable resource for students, medical professionals, patient support organizations, and anyone looking to obtain up-to-date cancer prevention information.

# 1

## CANCER AND ITS RISK FACTORS

The conclusion is that prevention is an effective way to reduce the risk of cancer. Everyone needs to be aware of the potential risks associated with their lifestyle choices and take preventative measures whenever possible. Increasing knowledge on early detection, making sure to perform preventative examinations, and eating a balanced, nutritious diet are all highly effective ways to reduce the risk of developing this deadly disease. Taking preventative action is essential to lowering the incidence of cancer in our society.

The conclusion that can be drawn is that prevention is one of the best strategies to reduce the risk of cancer. Prevention ranges from simple preventive measures, such as quitting smoking and avoiding excessive sun exposure, to lifestyle adjustments, such as eating healthily and exercising regularly. The importance of prevention cannot be stressed enough, particularly for those at high risk of developing cancer. Despite advances in cancer research and treatment, the vast majority of cancers are still preventable.

Prevention strategies that work at the population level must ultimately be harmonized into integrated and multi-sector approaches. These approaches should be combined with public health interventions to ensure the adoption of evidence-based, effective primary prevention strategies at the individual level. Local strategies that reduce exposure in areas with a high frequency of environmental contaminants must also be considered.

Cancer prevention must become an essential part of later health services offered at government and non-government health facilities. Patients should be provided with easy-to-understand information about cancer prevention to help them reduce their risk.

Efforts must also be made to strengthen national capabilities for cancer prevention, for example, by developing cancer registries and establishing dedicated research initiatives that help to inform prevention efforts.

To be able to make prevention and control strategies more effective, the root causes, the etiologies, and the risk factors for cancer need to be clearly identified and widely understood. For this purpose, government and community organizations need to specifically allocate resources for conducting population-based studies, encouraging awareness campaigns, and using innovative health promotion policies. Through these preventive measures, it may help to lower the risk of cancer not just in the individual, but on a large scale as well.

With concerted efforts, it is possible to substantially reduce the large disease burden associated with cancer in the future. Further research is needed on individual, societal, and regional patterns of cancer risk, in addition to examining the development and effectiveness of interventions. Well-targeted initiatives can make a positive impact that strengthens cancer prevention, control, and care efforts around the world.

# 2

## DETECTION OF CANCER AND AWARENESS

Being aware of the signs and symptoms of certain cancers can save a lot of lives. Cancer is a life-threatening disease that affects millions of people around the world. Despite many advancements in cancer detection, awareness is still lacking and it is essential to increase public knowledge about this devastating illness.

Early detection of cancer means that the chance of successful treatment is greater and that patients have better survival rates. It is important to recognize the physical indicators of cancer such as changes in skin color, unusual lumps or bumps, and unusual bleeding or discharge. However, these signs may not always appear in every type of cancer. A thorough screening can alert the patient to the possibility of cancer and refer them to a specialist to receive a diagnosis.

Cancer screening can be performed through a variety of methods. Physical exams of various organs can help note changes in the body, allowing for early detection through the catchment of warning signs. Various laboratory tests have also been developed to detect cancer, including screening for particular proteins or genetic changes. The process of testing for these changes helps a doctor determine if abnormal cells are present and diagnose a patient's risk for developing cancer.

Patients need to stay in tune and aware of their bodies and pay close attention to any changes that could potentially indicate the presence of cancer. If cancer is suspected, patients should consult their doctor for tests to definitive diagnose the condition. Depending on what symptoms a patient is experiencing and other risk factors that they might have, testing procedures such as X-rays, magnetic resonance imaging (MRI), or computed tomography (CT) may be recommended. For certain cancers, such as breast cancer, screening using a mammogram or counseling a patient to examine their bodies is integral for detection.

When it comes to cancer, it is important to remember that prevention and early diagnosis can make a huge difference in a patient's survival and prognosis rate. There are a variety of campaigns to raise awareness and support for detecting cancer at its earliest possible stages. As more individuals become active in the cancer-awareness movement, more lives can be saved.

# 3

## UNDERSTANDING HOW YOUR ENVIRONMENT AND BEHAVIORS CAN AFFECT YOUR RISK

The term "cancer" evokes strong emotion and unease because of its connection to life-altering illnesses. Although it can be frightening for people to consider, understanding how one's lifestyle and environment can affect their cancer risk is important.

Environmental factors such as exposure to radiation, chemicals, and unsafe drinking water can all increase your risk of developing cancer or cancer metastasis. However, the largest contributors to cancer risk are behavioral factors. The way that we live and the foods that we eat play a significant role in influencing our cancer risk.

Smoking tobacco, consistent exposure to second-hand smoke, and the use of smokeless products have been identified as leading causes of cancer. This is largely due to the carcinogenic chemicals they contain. It's important to remember that all areas of smoking have an associated level of risk. Cutting back even slightly on the frequency of smoking or using hand-rolled rather than manufactured cigarettes often has health benefits.

Along with tobacco products, overusing alcohol (defined on a daily/weekly basis), as well as poor sleeping habits, BMI, and diet are associated with increased risk as well. The typical Western diet is high in saturated/unsaturated fats and processed junk foods, and low in vegetables, leafy greens, and un/low-fat proteins – and this kind of diet is linked to imbalances in the body that can severely influence health and the potential for cancer.

Because chronic inflammation is associated with higher rates of cancer, it is incredibly important to focus on non-inflammatory nutrition. Foods that can trigger inflammation are fried, oily, and sugary foods, as well as meats that are very high in nitrates. To counteract chronic inflammation, try to include more healthy fats, proteins, fresh fruits and vegetables, and water as part of your diet. Taking active steps to manage one's stress and emotional health can benefit their overall health and coping with life events is also beneficial in this regard as well.

The influence between the atmosphere and everyday behavior on developing cancer is complex. While some factors like delayed pregnancy choices and the risk of HPV/hepatitis B transmission aren't entirely controllable, changing certain habits and maintaining a healthy lifestyle are great ways to look after one's well-being. Ultimately, cancer can be a changeable risk if one takes active steps in improving their lifestyle and eliminate any potential unhealthy habits.

# 4

## LIFESTYLE HABITS THAT CAN HELP REDUCE CANCER RISK

Living a healthy lifestyle is critical for reducing the risk of many diseases, including cancer. Some of the lifestyle Habits associated with a lower risk of developing cancer are listed here.

1.  Maintaining a Healthy Weight: Being overweight or obese is associated with a higher risk for many cancers, including colorectal, gastric, pancreatic, and postmenopausal breast cancer. Eating a diet high in fiber, fruits, and vegetables, and avoiding processed junk and fried foods can prevent men and women from becoming overweight.

2. Consuming Alcohol Moderately: Having more than one alcoholic drink per day for women and more than two per day for men may lead to higher cancer risk. Moderate drinking consists of no more than one drink per country for women and two for men, and individuals who don't drink should not start just to try and lower their cancer risk.

3. Participating in Regular Exercise: Exercise can benefit both physical and mental health, and may help reduce the

risk of cancer. Working out for at least 30 minutes per day on five or more days a week can help towards keeping a healthy weight, which as previously mentioned, can reduce cancer risk.

4. Limiting Sun Exposure: Spending too much time in the sun or tanning beds can increase the risk of skin cancer. Wearing sunscreen, covering up, and avoiding the direct sun between 10 am 12 and 4 pm can help reduce the risk of skin cancer.

5. Quitting Smoking: Smoking cigarettes has been linked to an increased risk of certain cancers - lung cancer being the most obvious one. Quitting smoking and avoiding secondhand smoke or vaping can greatly reduce cancer risk as well as improve one's overall health.

Living a healthy lifestyle can help to reduce the risk of developing cancer, though it cannot guarantee prevention. All individuals should visit their doctor and undergo regular screenings so that any changes in their health can be detected as soon as possible. Doing so can help one catch and treat an illness as early as possible, dramatically improving chances of recovery. Overall, important lifestyle habits such as exercise, consuming a balanced diet, not smoking, and limiting sun exposure are integral to helping decrease one's cancer risk.

# 5

## STRESS AND CANCER

Cancer is a term that can trigger feelings of fear and apprehension. Over the years, research has gained valuable insight into the causes of cancer and what treatments are available for its various forms, but stress remains one of the most likely contributors to certain types of cancer. Stress is particularly linked to certain types of cancer, and its diverse range of psychological and physiological effects can, directly and indirectly, influence the development of cancer cells. In this article, we explore how stress can contribute to cancer and list a few things people can do to manage their stress levels more effectively.

Stress is a natural byproduct of everyday life. Whether you're dealing with the pressures of work, managing family responsibilities, or coping with difficult events, it can be easy to become overwhelmed and let your stress take over. This, In turn, can put extra strain on our body's natural defense systems and make it harder for us to fight illness and disease; including cancer.

Stress has been linked to almost every type of cancer, but it's most commonly linked to certain ones such as breast cancer and colorectal cancer. The most common theory for this link is that, when a person experiences stress, their body produces too much cortisol which is a hormone released in response to stress. When levels of cortisol are too high, studies have suggested it can affect the progression of some cancers. Further, psychological and emotional factors caused by stress can have an indirect effect on the development of cancer. If your stress levels are abnormally high and not managed, then you're more likely to feel down and negative which can disrupt the functions of your body's immune system and impair its ability to fight the disease.

Whilst the connection between stress and cancer is one that is still being studied, there are a few things you can do to help protect yourself against further exacerbating this link. Some of the simple tips for managing stress include taking regular breaks and talking to family and friends as well as getting more sleep. Remembering to look after yourself and practicing relaxation techniques such as guided meditation or mindful yoga, can work wonders in reducing your overall stress levels and can be a great preventative measure against cancer.

Understanding the connection between stress and cancer can help us to be more aware of how we're managing our stress levels and take the appropriate steps to manage them more effectively. Taking a holistic approach to our stress management and engaging in calming activities daily can help create a healthier environment both mentally and physically, ultimately giving us more hope and strength for seeking higher chances of survival if and when the time comes for treating a cancer diagnosis.

It is a well-known fact that there is a definitive link between stress and your overall health – both physical and mental. Studies have revealed an increase in stress shown to be tied to a higher risk of developing certain types of cancer. While there currently is not a complete understanding of how stress impacts someone's chances of developing cancer, there are clear risk factors and possible contributions that can increase the chances of developing a serious health condition.

When a person is under a great amount of stress, regardless of the cause, their bodies restore balance by releasing a hormone called cortisol. Over time, the constant presence of cortisol might slowly start to make its way into the bloodstream. Studies have suggested the presence of high blood cortisol within the body may increase a person's chances of developing certain types of cancer.

Hormones, like cortisol, may be considered a stress role in the development of cancer in two different ways. In more aggressive and fast-moving types of cancer, cortisol creates something of a fuel source, helping to encourage uncontrolled growth at a faster speed than normal. On the opposite side of the spectrum, cortisol acts like cement for more passive types of cancer making them slow-growing but possibly harder to spot and diagnose until it's progressed to a more advanced stage.

It is important to note that there are many various causes of cancer and that although possible, stress alone doesn't always cause cancer by its nature. In cases that can generally be seen as high-stress events, like the formation of a cancerous tumor or some kind of hormone-enabled condition, cortisol levels may be at their highest moments. Though common sources of stress can come with divorce, PTSD, emotional trauma, etc – none of these particular events directly correlate with the development of cancer, which should not be used as a reason to still identify and manage your stress.

# 6

## EXCHANGE HARMFUL BEHAVIORS FOR HEALTH-PROMOTING CHOICES

The benefits of a healthy lifestyle are profound, and research continues to show that one of the most effective ways to promote health and reduce the risk of cancer is to make conscious choices regarding your behavior and lifestyle. In particular, replacing harmful behaviors with health-promoting choices is an essential factor in cancer prevention.

Leading a sedentary lifestyle or engaging in unhealthy activities can have alarming effects. Rich diets high in junk food, foods that are cooked at high temperatures, individual behaviors such as smoking cigarettes or excessive consumption of alcoholic beverages, lack of exercise, unprotected exposure to the sun, and exposure to certain threats at home and in the environment are all known cancer risk factors.

Fortunately, there are many effective strategies to promote health and reduce the risk of cancer, and it starts with recognizing our tendencies and replacing them with healthier alternatives.

One of the most advantageous steps to start making healthy behaviors a regular part of your life is to adopt regular physical exercise. At least 30 minutes of exercise daily as well as maintaining an active lifestyle is not only beneficial to your physical well-being but also a great contributor to cancer prevention. Additionally, it has been found that staying lean and having a BMI less than 25 decreases the risk of cancer across the body.

A healthy diet also helps to combat cancer risk factors. Combining more plant-based foods like fresh fruits and vegetables, cereals, and grains can significantly improve your nutrition intake and help reduce your fat consumption. Additionally, increasing fiber intake promotes better digestion and can also decrease the risk of certain cancers, like Colorectal. Eating foods free from preservatives as well as thoroughly cooked proteins may also become instrumental in your fight against cancer.

Lastly, individuals must watch for behaviors that may increase cancer risk. Abstaining from the use of tobacco products, reducing sun exposure, and limiting alcoholic beverages may go a long way in cancer prevention. Also, be mindful of certain chemicals found in colored tattoos, household products, and makeup.

At the end of the day, making healthy choices in all aspects of your life is essential to reducing cancer risk factors. Small adjustments such as adopting regular physical exercise, consuming a healthier diet, limiting unhealthy behaviors, and making conscious decisions regarding unsafe habits all contribute to being beneficial for your health. Making sure you are conscious of harmful behaviors is an essential step in preventing and preparing for potential cancer.

# 7

## USE OF SUPPLEMENTS AND FUNCTIONAL FOODS IN CANCER RISK REDUCTION

We know that a healthy diet is important to support the physical health of individuals. It is especially pertinent to know the different types of healthy food available that can act as cancer-preventive agents. Nutritionists are constantly emphasizing using supplements and functional foods for reducing the risk of cancer.

Supplements like antioxidants, vitamins, and minerals are used to arm our bodies against cancer. Antioxidants such as Vitamin C, Vitamin E, carotenoids, carotenoids, and polyphenols stop our cells from experiencing oxidative stress, which can increase cancer risk.

In terms of vitamins, folate (a form of vitamin B-9) is often used as a supplement for reducing the risk of certain cancers. Research has generally found that the use of folate may reduce the risk of several types of cancer, including colorectal cancer. Additionally, Vitamin D supplementation offers protection against the progression of breast cancer.

Minerals have also been shown to help fight cancer. Selenium functions as an antioxidant, which can help protect against cancer-causing agents in the environment.

Selenium, when combined with Vitamin C and Vitamin E, can provide additional protection.

Foods that are naturally rich in bioactive compounds are known as "functional foods". They are known to offer greater health benefits than traditional foods and include probiotics, ginger, and green tea.

Probiotics, or live microorganisms in the form of yogurts, reduce the risk of gut-related cancers, especially those linked to colorectal cancer. Likewise, ginger is also known for offering even greater protection as it has very strong anti-inflammatory properties. This makes it an effective anti-cancer ingredient in our bodies.

Studies have also concluded that green tea may offer protection against the risk of cancer. Tea is known to contain polyphenols that can prevent lung and oral cancer.

In summary, the use of supplements and functional food is essential in maintaining our physical health and in preventing certain types of cancer. Integrating food items that contain the aforementioned substances can work wonders for our bodies. Therefore, keep conscious of the dietary choices you make and pay specific focus to keeping cancer as far away as possible.

# 8

## PHYSICAL ACTIVITY AND EXERCISE AS CANCER PREVENTION

Cancer is an uncontrolled growth of cells that can spread quickly and become dangerous to our health. Regular physical activity and exercise can be powerful tools in helping to prevent cancer.

We know that regular exercise can reduce the risk of several types of cancers, including bowel, breast, endometrial, and colon cancer. While the exact cause and effect are still being studied, many believe the mechanisms which produce these results can be attributed to the decrease in body fat that many people who exercise regularly experience. Proper bodily activity has long been associated with the prevention of chronic diseases, however, the effects of activity on cancer have only recently been studied in depth.

One way physical activity helps to reduce cancer can be attributed to calorie control. When exercising regularly, the body is kept active – meaning the body burns more calories and prevents weight gain. Being overweight or obese is linked to various forms of cancer, including kidney cancer. Studies suggest a direct correlation between greater degrees of obesity and increased cases of cancer, while regular physical activity may help to maintain a healthy weight and, in turn, ward off cancer.

Other studies suggest that physical activity can protect the body against hormone-related cancers, as regular exercise helps to balance hormones and prevent them from harming the body. Exercise also works to improve the body's immune system – a stronger immune system increases the body's ability to fight off cardiovascular disease, cancer, and other maladies. In turn, it has been postulated that those with a stronger immune system could be at less risk for developing cancer.

We all know that physical activity has benefits for overall health in the form of improved cardiovascular system, improved respiratory system, and better muscular endurance, but now research is showing its effects on cancer prevention too. And while we don't yet have definitive proof that regular exercise can curb cancer, the evidence is there to suggest that exercise acts as a buffer against the disease. So, get moving today and lower your cancer risk!

Physical activity and exercise can be an important preventative measure against many types of cancer, primarily through its positive effect on a person's overall health. Exercise is known to help maintain a healthy weight, reduce stress, and decrease a person's risk for high blood pressure, diabetes, and heart disease, and has now been linked to decreasing the odds of getting diagnosed with cancer.

For cancer prevention, the World Health Organization recommends adults ages 18-64 should do at least 150 minutes of moderate-intensity activity per week or 75 minutes of vigorous-intensity aerobic activity. Additionally, to gain some beneficial health effects, it's suggested that adults do twice the amount that is recommended or 300 minutes of moderate-intensity exercise per week. Getting aerobic and strengthening activities every week can produce even more powerful health benefits and further decrease the risk of being diagnosed with cancer. It's key to exercise in a way that moves the entire body, engaging the legs, arms, and hips – swimming, running, and brisk walking can all be great options.

Recent studies conducted on colon and breast cancer survivors attest to the effectiveness of physical activity in long-term survivorship; those who have been physically active for at least one hour a day in their lifetime – leading up to and post-diagnosis, were less likely to have recurrences years further on. More research suggests people part of a program combining diet, exercise, stress reduction, and lifestyle change are also more likely several years out to have much more cancer-free survival than people will participate only in physical activity.

It's estimated one half to two-thirds of deaths due to bladder, breast, colon, liver, endometrial and other cancers are partially preventable by physical activity and exercise. While it's regulated closely, studies are also being conducted to see if aerobic exercise can further help individuals undergoing treatments to lessen side effects from whatever therapy they are using.

Adopting a healthy lifestyle including a routine of physical activity is key for reducing any chances of having cancer; however, the process must be reasonable and realistic for it to be successful. So, consult your doctor if you're at increased of being diagnosed with cancer, and together develop a lifestyle plan that suits what you can physically handle without overworking yourself and improve your chances of living a healthy lifestyle.

# 9

## MAINTAINING A HEALTHY BODY WEIGHT AND IMPROVING YOUR DIET

Leading an active lifestyle and maintaining a healthy body weight are essential components of cancer prevention. Being overweight or obese increases the risk of several types of cancer, including breast cancer, colon cancer, and uterine cancer. By eating a healthy diet and exercising regularly, you can reduce your risk of cancer and improve your overall health.

In this chapter, we will explore how to maintain a healthy body weight, which foods to incorporate into your diet for better health, and how to incorporate physical activities into your lifestyle to benefit your health and reduce your risk of cancer.

To effectively maintain a healthy body weight, you should practice mindful eating. Make sure to eat slowly so that diet-busting cravings don't creep up. Snack on healthy foods in between meals and try to avoid processed foods with added sugar or trans-fats. Instead, choose to snack on fruits, vegetables, nuts, and seeds - all of which contain essential vitamins, minerals, and fiber. Also ensure your complete your meals with balanced diets full of healthy fats, proteins, whole grains, and fiber, rather than consuming processed foods and meals full of saturated fat and sugar.

Incorporating more whole, nourishing foods into your diet can support healthy body weight as well as reduce the risk of related health problems such as cancer. Whole grains, lean proteins, legumes, nuts, and seeds, and fresh foods like fruits and vegetables are beneficial for overall health and also improve tolerance when eating varied healthy foods. Incorporating seasonal vegetables, as well as more variety within each meal, is also beneficial to help ensure all your nutritional needs are met. Additionally, adding herbs and spices to food helps boost flavor and provide more health advantages due to their antioxidant compounds.

Exercising regularly and engaging in physical activities like running, walking, cycling, and swimming can also help maintain a healthy weight and provide psychological benefits. Activities can also involve gardening, playing, yoga, and tai chi, as well as household chores. For cancer prevention purposes, combining aerobic exercises and muscular strength can help patients get more benefits.

In summary, maintaining healthy body weight and improving your diet should be included as part of your cancer prevention plan. The benefits of making these changes to your lifestyle can not only reduce the risk of cancer but can improve all aspects of your physical and mental health. Eating whole and nourishing ingredients and engaging in regular physical activities can set up an environment conducive to decreased cancer risk.

# 10

## CANCER SCREENINGS - WHAT TO EXPECT AND WHEN

Cancer screenings are vital for early detection and diagnosis, increasing the chances of successful treatment and possibly a cure. These routine check-ups have become the gold standard in preventive health and are recommended to keep you on top of your potential cancer risk. Knowing what to expect when you go and when you should be sure to go are just a few aspects of understanding the screening process as recommended by your healthcare provider.

### Types of Screenings

Depending on your medical history, age, and gender, your doctor may recommend one or a variety of screening tests. Your typical screening test may include prostate exams, mammograms, pelvic exams, and colonoscopies. It is important to know the warning signs associated with any type of cancer to recognize when a visit to the doctor is necessary.

### When It Should Be Done

Cancer screenings become more frequent as you age, which is why your doctor may recommend a different frequency for your tests. A routine colonoscopy may be recommended every 5-10 years. A cervical exam, like a Pap test, may happen every two years. A mammogram should typically be done annually after 40. There is also the option of a blood screening, which looks for the presence of biochemical markers. This type of test helps indicate the possibility of cancerous cells.

**What to Expect**

Before screening starts, the doctor will ask about your medical history and family history. You'll likely give blood for lab work and have a physical exam. Depending on the test or tests you are having, you may also get an internal exam or receive ultrasound images of your body.

The results from the screening and the response from your doctor should be discussed. If no cancer is found, your doctor may recommend preventative measures or additional tests and screenings based on test results and to further monitor risk factors. If cancer is found, you will be referred to a specialist and begin making a plan of action to best approach your diagnosis.

Overall, cancer screenings are important to detect, prevent, and possibly cure cancer. It is important to be aware of the benefits and challenges that screenings may bring to properly approach any test or potential diagnosis. Be sure to discuss screenings with your doctor to determine when they should be done; which tests are best for you; and what type of preventative lifestyle Risk reduction strategies should be implemented.

# 11

## MINORITIES AND CANCER OCCURRENCE

Cancer is a widespread illness, which can affect all populations across the globe. Minority populations living in financially or medically underserved areas, often experience specific risk factors and educational obstacles associated with cancer occurrences and education to prevent them. Higher rates of poverty, disease, and higher rates of overall health illiteracy are all concerning issues facing minorities when it comes to things such as cancer awareness and treatments.

Cancer occurrence in minorities is an issue as different types of cancer are drastically more common in specific minority groups. Hispanic, African American, and certain East Asian populations are all at a greater risk for certain forms of cancer, such as colorectal, cervical, and prostate cancer. These higher rates result from a combination of higher risk factors, such as certain lifestyle habits that are common amongst a particular ethnic group and economic disadvantages which limit the ability of minorities to access disease prevention resources, such as cancer screenings.

It's incredibly important that when people think about cancer occurrence in minorities, the more unique factors related to being a minority become important considerations for prevention and treatment services. Understanding the shared risk feelings, cultural norms, and values relating to cancer occurrences might help explain why some might be more or less likely to go for preventative health care or self-perceived painful or embarrassing screenings. Additionally, language barriers can further contribute to the disproportionate use of healthcare resources by these vulnerable populations.

Access to public and private insurance has been shown to play a major role in determining colon cancer prevention and treatment stratagems for minorities. Even amongst those that potentially qualify, many minorities may not be educated in pursuing those paths or may not trust their validity. If communities, health providers, and organizations wish to proactively produce lower rates of cancer among minorities, innovative health outreach programs, such as free health education classes and culturally tailored health agencies need to be incorporated to bridge these knowledge and confidence gaps.

Cancer continues to be a concerning subject for minorities, on multiple levels. Programs that target public education, higher access to resources, and more streamlined client/patient options could help to reduce cancer occurrence rates and aid desirable innovations in procedural treatments. With proactive strategies on being more understanding and inclusive of individual minority challenges, solving the underlying causes of an unequal health system divided by race can become a reality.

# 12

## SUPPORT AND COPING STRATEGIES AFTER A CANCER DIAGNOSIS

Cancer is the leading cause of death globally and is a diagnosis that can be overwhelming to many. After you have received a diagnosis of cancer, the next steps can seem complicated. To optimize your health during treatment, it is important to have a plan for taking the necessary steps for support and coping strategies to cope with the diagnosis. This article will provide an overview of support and coping strategies that can be used after a cancer diagnosis.

### Types of Support

The primary forms of support for people after a cancer diagnosis include self-care, medicines, surgery, radiation, and support from family and friends. All these forms of emotional, social, and spiritual support are essential after a cancer diagnosis.

**Self-care** includes actions that reduce the physical, emotional, or mental stress associated with cancer. This can be done by learning the facts about cancer, talking with a healthcare provider, having a balanced diet, exercising regularly, getting enough rest, and finding ways to relax. Additionally, maintaining rituals and routines such as keeping a journal, practicing meditation, and deep breathing exercises can contribute to creating a sense of meaning and control through the process.

**Medicines** are one of the most common forms of support for a person with cancer. Depending on the type of cancer, medicine can be used to reduce tumor size, maintain hormone balance, reduce inflammation or pain, or manage other side effects. It is important to talk to your doctor about what medications to take, what the risks are, and how the treatments may affect your lifestyle.

**Surgery, radiation, and chemotherapy** are specialized treatments for certain kinds of cancer. Surgery is used to remove a tumor, which can be partial or complete, or reconstruct a body part affected by cancer. Radiation and chemotherapy can be extremely effective treatments in targeting abnormal cells and eliminating the potential for the recurrence of cancer or metastasis to other parts of the body. It is important to talk to your doctor about the specific treatment and any potential side effects.

**Family and friends** also provide a tremendous level of support for a person after a cancer diagnosis. For many people, talking with family and friends about the diagnosis is an essential part of coping with the news. Additionally, family and friends are an invaluable resource for providing emotional and practical help.

## Coping Strategies

When facing a cancer diagnosis, it is important to have a plan to cope with the uncertainty, fear, and anxiety associated with it. This includes developing healthy habits to manage stress, understanding the available information about your type of cancer, researching different treatment options, maintaining relationships with family and friends, managing emotions, and getting proper rest.

Developing healthy coping skills is important when dealing with cancer. Examples of healthy coping include mindful relaxation, progressive muscle relaxation, journaling, light exercise, eating healthfully with nutritious meals, and getting a good night's sleep. Talking with a supportive person (such as a close family member, friend, or mental health professional) to discuss any fears or worries can also be helpful.

Learning about the type of cancer and collecting information about different treatment methods will help you make informed decisions about your treatment. Reading advice books on cancer and the experiences of fellow patients can help you identify strategies for coping with cancer. Additionally, talking with a medical professional about the cancer, side effects from treatment, and expectations from treatment is important.

Maintaining your relationships with family, friends, and colleagues is essential when it comes to coping with a cancer diagnosis. Even though talking with others may be emotionally draining, it is important to seek help from people who can provide emotional and practical support when you need it. Additionally, establishing meaningful connections and networks can provide social support when coping with the diagnosis.

Expressing and managing emotions can be difficult when living with cancer. Negative emotions, such as fear, anger, and helplessness, can become overwhelming and difficult to manage. To best cope with these negative emotions, it is essential to take active steps for managing stress, such as meditation or other relaxation techniques, listening to music, watching favorite movies, talking with supportive individuals, and writing in a journal.

Finally, getting ample rest is essential when facing a cancer diagnosis. Aim for 7-9 hours of sleep and make sure the quality of sleep is sound. Creating a comfortable environment to rest in is also important in terms of darkness, quietness, cool temperature, and relaxed breathing. Pursuing certain activities before bedtime such as decreasing screen time and engaging in calming activities can help foster restful sleep.

Above all, people living with cancer need to focus on their self-care. Prioritize activities and habits that will help take care of your mental and emotional health as well as your physical health to best cope with a cancer diagnosis. Additionally, talking with your healthcare team, practicing healthy coping mechanisms, connecting with supportive family and friends, and getting proper rest are all critical elements of recovering from a cancer diagnosis.

# 13

## CONCLUSION - PREVENTION CAN REDUCE THE RISK OF CANCER

The conclusion is that prevention is an effective way to reduce the risk of cancer. Everyone needs to be aware of the potential risks associated with their lifestyle choices and take preventative measures whenever possible. Increasing knowledge on early detection, making sure to perform preventative examinations, and eating a balanced, nutritious diet are all highly effective ways to reduce the risk of developing this deadly disease. Taking preventative action is essential to lowering the incidence of cancer in our society.

The conclusion that can be drawn is that prevention is one of the best strategies to reduce the risk of cancer. Prevention ranges from simple preventive measures, such as quitting smoking and avoiding excessive sun exposure, to lifestyle adjustments, such as eating healthily and exercising regularly. The importance of prevention cannot be stressed enough, particularly for those at high risk of developing cancer. Despite advances in cancer research and treatment, the vast majority of cancers are still preventable.

Prevention strategies that work at the population level must ultimately be harmonized into integrated and multi-sector approaches. These approaches should be combined with public health interventions to ensure the adoption of evidence-based, effective primary prevention strategies at the individual level. Local strategies that reduce exposure in areas with a high frequency of environmental contaminants must also be considered.

Cancer prevention must become an essential part of later health services offered at government and non-government health facilities. Patients should be provided with easy-to-understand information about cancer prevention to help them reduce their risk.

Efforts must also be made to strengthen national capabilities for cancer prevention, for example, by developing cancer registries and establishing dedicated research initiatives that help to inform prevention efforts.

To be able to make prevention and control strategies more effective, the root causes, the etiologies, and the risk factors for cancer need to be clearly identified and widely understood. For this purpose, government and community organizations need to specifically allocate resources for conducting population-based studies, encouraging awareness campaigns, and using innovative health promotion policies. Through these preventive measures, it may help to lower the risk of cancer not just in the individual, but on a large scale as well.

With concerted efforts, it is possible to substantially reduce the large disease burden associated with cancer in the future. Further research is needed on individual, societal, and regional patterns of cancer risk, in addition to examining the development and effectiveness of interventions. Well-targeted initiatives can make a positive impact that strengthens cancer prevention, control, and care efforts around the world.

# ABOUT THE AUTHOR

I specialize in self-help, health and fitness writing. I have been passionate about health and wellness for all of my life and helping others pursue healthier, happier, and more satisfying lives is what motivates me daily. I love to dive into health and fitness topics to help readers connect with the material in a more personal way. As a long-time personal trainer, group fitness instructor, and healthy lifestyle advocate I feel that I have the knowledge and experience to share tips, stories, and insights. As an inspiring motivator, I empower my readers and help them live an active, fulfilling life.